# Playing God

**Also compiled from** *Tabletalk*

*Doubt and Assurance*
*Vanity and Meaning*

# Playing God

Dissecting Biomedical Ethics
and Manipulating the Body

Edited by

# R. C. Sproul Jr.

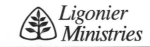
Ligonier
Ministries

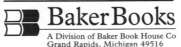
BakerBooks
A Division of Baker Book House Co
Grand Rapids, Michigan 49516

©1997 by Ligonier Ministries

Published by Baker Books
a division of Baker Book House Company
P.O. Box 6287, Grand Rapids, MI 49516-6287

Printed in the United States of America

For information about academic books, resources for Christian leaders, and all new releases available from Baker Book House, visit our web site:
http://www.bakerbooks.com

Library of Congress Cataloging-in-Publication Data

Playing God : dissecting biomedical ethics and manipulating the body / edited by R. C. Sproul, Jr.
    p. cm.
    ISBN 0-8010-5725-6 (pbk.)
    1. Medical ethics. 2. Christian ethics. I. Sproul, R. C. (Robert Craig), 1965–.
R725.56.P56  1997
174'.2—dc20                                                    96-35213

The material contained in this book was published originally in *Tabletalk* magazine and was compiled in this format by the editor of *Tabletalk*, R. C. Sproul Jr.

# Contents

# Contributors

*Michael S. Beates,* dean of students at Reformed Theological Seminary, Orlando, Florida.

*Harold O. J. Brown,* professor of biblical and systematic theology at Trinity Evangelical Divinity School, Deerfield, Illinois, and chairman of the Christian Action Council.

*Nigel M. de S. Cameron,* associate dean of academic doctoral programs at Trinity Evangelical Divinity School, Deerfield, Illinois, and editor of the journal *Ethics and Medicine.*

*Kenneth L. Connor,* trial lawyer in Tallahassee, Florida, past chairman of the State of Florida Commission on Ethics, currently vice chairman of Americans United for Life.

*Randy Crenshaw, M.D.,* medical director of Humana Health Care Plans of Alabama.

*George Grant,* director of The King's Meadow Study Center in Franklin, Tennessee.

*W. Andrew Hoffecker,* professor of religion at Grove City College, Pennsylvania.

*Mike Malone,* pastor of St. Paul's Presbyterian Church (PCA), Orlando, Florida.

*J. P. Moreland,* director of the M.A. program in apologetics and professor of philosophy at Talbot School of Theology, La Mirada, California.

*Ken Myers*, host of *Mars Hill Tapes,* an audiotape magazine on Christianity and culture.

*R. C. Sproul,* chairman of Ligonier Ministries and teacher on the national radio program *Renewing Your Mind.*

*R. C. Sproul Jr.,* director of The Highlands Study Center in Meadowview, Virginia, and editor of *Tabletalk.*

*Part 1*

# Dissecting Medical Ethics

Soldiers were dying. Lands that once conjured images of sandy beaches, swaying palms, and sunshine became bloody battle-fields: Pearl Harbor, Coral Sea, Iwo Jima. As courageous men assaulted beachheads and landing strips, a second battle raged, a battle of wits. Scientists, unaccustomed to the crude tools of war, set their minds to a pinpoint, focusing on the most basic of elements. The Manhattan Project sought to harness the power of matter and bring a swift end to World War II. The war was over the issue of rulership, who would have dominion over the planet. It was settled by who first gained dominion over the atom.

This is the essence of science: the attempt to wield dominion over nature. It is a noble venture, at the very core of God's first command to man: "Be fruitful and increase in number; fill the earth and subdue it. Rule over the fish of the sea and the birds of the air and over every living creature that moves on the ground" (Gen. 1:28). The dominion to which Adam and Eve were called was not absolute. They remained accountable to their Creator until the fall. In eating of the tree, they sought ultimate authority and gave no heed to their Maker.

Science and the subduing of the earth continue. We take for granted our conquest. Mankind has moved from traveling on foot to harnessing the power of animals to soaring through the skies to planting a flag on the moon. Since the fall, however, the noble work of science has been tainted with the ignoble. Science devoid of the authority of God is an attempt to wield his dominion.

We are exploring biomedical ethics, in which science touches upon life itself. We are witnesses to increasing wonders of healing. Illnesses once deemed fatal are now mere temporary inconveniences. Euthanasia, abortion, gene manipulation, *in vitro* fertilization, and issues still to come present an unprecedented ethical challenge to the thoughtful Christian. As always our technical prowess is testing the limits of our wisdom. We find ourselves walking the razor's edge between life and death, between dominion and rebellion.

We are called to continue to progress as we subdue the earth. We must do so, however, *coram Deo*, before the face of God, recognizing and bowing before his authority over us. We are to rule his creation, remembering that "the earth is the LORD's and all that is in it" (Ps. 24:1 NRSV). We can never forget that we are of the earth we seek to rule. From the earth he fashioned us and so made us his own. We are commanded to seek his directive and his wisdom as we confront these most complex issues.

# Healing, Suffering, and the New Medicine

*Nigel M. de S. Cameron*

Behind the battles being fought over abortion and behind the insidious threat of euthanasia, a struggle is underway for the very soul of medicine. Abortion and euthanasia, like the crises in health-care costs and resourcing, are symptoms; they are not the disease. Treating symptoms has always been part of the physician's duty, but unless the patient is incurable, it is never the most important duty.

Behind these traumatic symptoms, what is *wrong* with medicine? Medicine used to be all about healing, if possible, and if not, treating symptoms and making a chronic or terminal condition as bearable as possible. Healing was the lead idea. Instead the key today is power. Medicine is now an exercise in power over the patient, the clinical situation an occasion of manipulation. Healing, of course, is still on the agenda, but it has been displaced as its first item, its defining characteristic. That is the real significance for the medicine of abortion, as the doctor turns technician and will either help bring the unborn child to term or kill the child in the womb—depending on his or her instructions from the mother (and an appropriate fee). It is the same thing with euthanasia, that strange negation of medicine in which the physician kills on request. The pressure to legalize this practice is strong in the United States, fueled by fear of bad medicine and a growing desire to control not just our medical care but life and death. The defeat of Proposition 161 in California on November 3, 1992, by no means signals the end of the argument: It has just begun. In Holland there has been widespread euthanasia for a decade, so we need to grasp that the threat it poses is not science fiction.

And let's be clear what we mean: Euthanasia, as practiced in Holland, is not withholding treatment but killing by injection or some similar method.

The introduction of killing— before and after birth—as an option open to the physician symbolizes the momentous change that has come in medicine. One way to visualize that change is as a consumeristic reduction of the relationship of patient and physician. Of course, there have always been parallels in commercial relationships. Doctors have usually (though, in the best medicine, not always) been paid fees for their services. Patients have generally been able to choose between doctors. But there has always been more to it. The

> *Medicine is now an exercise in power over the patient, the clinical situation an occasion of manipulation. Healing, of course, is still on the agenda, but it has been displaced as its first item, its defining characteristic.*

physician, once called in to see a patient, has an open-ended responsibility for that patient's well-being. She or he has in the past worked through that responsibility in the terms we have noted: healing if possible, treating symptoms if not. The notion that the physician is really attending to consumer wants is novel. Not only so, it is subverting the whole system of health care in opening the door to medical killing; for if medicine is consumer driven, death may be what the consumer wants.

Behind this reduction lies something else. Time and again we are told that the sanctity of life must be qualified by a concern to relieve suffering. The patient who no longer wishes to face the challenges of continued living should be allowed to find an easy way out. Suffering should be relieved by death. We note in passing that these arguments are gaining ground at the moment when our medical resources are greater than they have ever been (for all our problems in containing costs). In recent years we have seen amazing advances in drug therapies and the collection of skills associated with palliative care and hospice—care for the dying.

What do these changes mean? Let us first go back to gain a perspective, back to the origin of modern medicine that lies in a combination of Judeo-Christian values and the special medicine of Hippocrates from ancient, pagan Greece. Christians followed the Hippocratic pattern—the pattern of healing and service with which we have become so familiar—since it fit so well their Bible-based concern for human dignity, love for one another, disinterested service, and especially, the sanctity of life. Hippocrates rejected abortion and euthanasia, and the church endorsed this high professional standard as a context for the practice of Christian medicine.

The Hippocratic physician was committed to a special set of values. That commitment was public and left neither doctor nor patient with any choice on the fundamental matters other than what those values supported. Nothing more than healing was the physician's business. More important than the particular requirements of the Hippocratic Oath, a moral framework was set in place. That is, medicine from its modern origins in Hippocratic paganism had come to be defined in moral terms. It could not be reduced to skill and power and patient autonomy.

The contrast with the "consumer wants" model could hardly be greater, though in many cases the result may be the same because the consumer wants to be healed. Yet that is breaking down in two ways. First, as we have noted, the consumer may *not* want to be healed but to be killed. Secondly, the consumer and the patient may not be one and the same. That is plainly the case with abortion: The consumer is the mother, and the patient who is killed (to relieve the mother's "suffering") is someone else. But that is not the only example of this sinister transfer. One of the main practical objections to voluntary euthanasia is that it often will not be voluntary at all. Even if the patient is competent—so someone else is not simply making a decision on her behalf—her own choice may be subtly but deeply influenced by what her relatives want, what her doctor suggests, or what she *thinks* her relatives or the doctor want her to do. Anyone with elderly relatives knows from experience how hard it can be to sort out what they want from what they think you want them to want. Add the pressure of illness, attendant depression, and financial concerns and the problem can prove insoluble.

As the Dutch experience already has shown, many cases of euthanasia are not voluntary at all. The consumer who is making the decisions may not be the patient. The choice may be deeply influenced by insurers, health-care authorities, or the government, all of which may have an interest in a certain kind of decision because it will save money. They also may have many means at their disposal to pressure patients in that direction. Of whose suffering then do we speak? The Patient Self-Determination Act with its strong encouragement of (almost always cost-saving) living wills is as good an example as we could seek.

Against such a power play, in which the patient is typically the least powerful player, Christian Hippocratism set a fixed moral framework to which the patient was as committed as the physician. It is one of the curiosities of Western civilization that Hippocratism triumphed in the pagan world, was adopted by Christians, and remains the formal context for medicine even today (the oath often etched on the commencement programs of numerous medical schools). The breakup of this value tradition marks one of the most telling casualties in the decline of Christendom and is loaded with significance for much more than the professional practice of the medical elite.

What can we do? Our practical strategy in looking beyond issues like abortion to the ideological struggle taking place in the cockpit of medical and human values must be twofold. We must work to kindle and rekindle a Christian medical tradition, maintaining the best of Christian Hippocratism and preserving it as an increasingly alternative and marginalized medical culture. But we must not fall prey once more to the temptation to pull out of the world in a monastic withdrawal. Christian Hippocratism must become the base from which we advance and engage with the post-Hippocratic medical culture. We will offer a medicine of care and concern, stripped of the illusion of commercial analogy and reinvigorated with the philanthropism that has always motivated the best in our medical culture. And that will be not least among the gospel messages we preach.

# Of Doctors and Other Priests

*Michael S. Beates*

I admit it—I hate hospitals. Particular sounds, visual images, smells, and even certain fleeting tastes encountered by my senses drag me inexorably back to scenes in assorted hospitals. Over the past ten years, my elder daughter, Jessica, my wife, Mary, and I have weathered at least twelve hospitalizations, not including the birth of four children, numerous exams, procedures, and the gray-hair-producing emergency room excursions. Don't get me wrong, I am grateful for medical technology. It is likely that my daughter and I may not have survived certain afflictions without the benefits of modern medicine. So, like many, while I dislike much of the health-care experience, I also realize that at times my life depends on doctors as they employ their knowledge and skill to intercede between me and death.

Like most people, too often I live only in the realm of the here and now, forgetting the eternal dimension of our existence. Death is the enemy of this physical existence, and we elevate doctors to the status of modern-day high priests to ward off the foe. Because the pragmatic use of life-preserving technology has accelerated so rapidly, we have lost the moral ability to accept death as our forefathers did. Try as we might, "man is destined to die once" (Heb. 9:27). Biomedical technology, like all technologies, is a god that limps and, ultimately, is unable to save.

Because of this inevitability, it is imperative to think through how you will respond in the face of a personal or family health crisis. Medical ethics becomes a pressing issue at the least expected moments. Without five minutes of prior thought, people must make life and death decisions. Thus it is necessary to consider the issues before circumstances force you to face them. Though variables and complexities preclude arriving at specific, detailed responses, our understanding of the character of God and the principles of our faith must be primary elements of the grid through which all such decisions will pass. Because of the consequences, biomedical ethics is far too important to leave to doctors and health-care administrators.

The practice of transplanting tissue and organs has become so routine that new advances are barely noticed. But recently we have moved to a new threshold—using human tissue that requires the death of the donor (fetal tissue harvested from aborted children and organ transplants from anencephalic children). The case of "Baby Theresa" in Florida less than a year ago has resulted in proposed legislation in this state to legalize the taking of primary organs from such babies prior to their death, thus killing them. The proposed law contends these babies do not possess the status of full personhood deserving preservation, this despite the acknowledgment that anencephalic children are unique chromosomal human beings who can live (albeit ever so briefly) outside the womb.

As believers our bodies are the temple of the Holy Spirit, and we have a duty as stewards of the body to maintain our lives as long as we can. However, we can never do so at the expense of another human life, no matter how deformed that life may be in our eyes (see Exod. 4:10–11 where God takes credit for creating what we call handicaps, deformities, and disabilities). Believers who could extend their lives with such "cutting-edge" biomedical technology must be prepared by God's grace to refuse the "benefits" of ungodly technologies and face their earthly death with the

> *Biomedical technology, like all technologies, is a god that limps and, ultimately, is unable to save.*

assurance that "our light and momentary troubles are achieving for us an eternal glory that far outweighs them all. So we fix our eyes not on what is seen, but on what is unseen. For what is seen is temporary and what is unseen is eternal" (2 Cor. 4:17–18).

While medical doctors may act as modern high priests, there is only one true High Priest, the Author and Finisher of our faith, Christ Jesus. In Hebrews Jesus is clearly portrayed as the ultimate priest whose work makes obsolete all those who came before or followed after. He was made like us (Heb. 2:14, 17), has suffered beyond our suffering (2:10, 18; 4:15), and his priestly work is comprehensive (4:14; 7:24–26), redeeming body and soul for eternal life. It is a work that is perfect and complete, not lacking in anything (7:28).

Acknowledge your dependence on him for each and every breath. Determine (while your health abounds) that when health fails (and medical technologies also fail) you will, by his grace, not only live but also die *coram Deo*, before God, under his authority and in his tender priestly care.

There is no shortage of books addressing biomedical ethics, but I recommend among others the following:

Cameron, Nigel M. de S. *The New Medicine: Life and Death after Hippocrates*. Wheaton: Crossway Books, 1992.

Frame, John M. *Medical Ethics: Principles, Persons, and Problems*. Phillipsburg, N.J.: Presbyterian and Reformed Publishing, 1988.

Horan, Dennis J., and David Mall, eds. *Death, Dying, and Euthanasia*. Westport, Conn.: Greenwood Press, 1980.

Medina, John. *The Outer Limits of Life*. Nashville: Oliver-Nelson, 1991.

Orr, Robert D., et al. *Life and Death Decisions*. Colorado Springs: NavPress, 1990.

Tada, Joni Eareckson. *When Is It Right to Die? Suicide, Euthanasia, Suffering, Mercy*. Grand Rapids: Zondervan, 1992.

# Death with Dignity: The "Right" to Die

*Harold O. J. Brown*

According to an article which appeared in *The Statesman* (Great Britain) thirty years ago, "The abortion wave of the sixties will be the euthanasia wave of the eighties." Abortion on demand was legalized nationwide in the United States several years later than in the United Kingdom, and therefore our abortion wave came in the seventies. A euthanasia wave, it seems, is rolling in right on schedule, twenty years later.

The term euthanasia, literally "good" or "happy" death, was used in the sixteenth century to refer to a death at peace with God and man, with the benefit of "ghostly counsel" (spiritual ministry), without undue suffering, and in the confidence of eternal life. For stoically inclined Greeks and Romans, a happy death was an honorable death, more often than not on the battlefield. The Vikings sought to be preserved from what they called a straw death—dying in bed rather than in heroic combat.

The Darwinian evolution revolution made millions of individuals and much of society forget that we human beings—men, women, and children, healthy or infirm, brilliant or simple— are all made in the image of God. Instead, it took for granted that we are in all essentials like the "other animals," the products of matter plus time, space, and chance. Bereft of anything that could be called a deathless soul, and with no prospect of a resurrection to eternal life, a man's existence seemed to have value and meaning only as long as it served the interests of others and made sense to the man himself.

In classical pagan antiquity, it was more or less taken for granted that human beings have the right to kill themselves. The reform movement in medicine, associated with the name of Hippocrates, the "father of medicine," followed the teaching of the philosopher Pythagoras, holding that we are made in the image of the divine, repudiating suicide, and making aspiring physicians vow never to participate in or encourage it.

*The sugar on euthanasia is largely semantic: The terms death with dignity and right to die have made it progressively easier to swallow.*

Euthanasia began to be a widely discussed option in Christendom in the aftermath of World War I. At first, its advocates were quite frank about what they meant by the word, calling it mercy killing. Because Hitler had an overt euthanasia program—a foretaste of his later enterprise of genocide—the term and the practice plummeted in popularity and social acceptability during the late 1930s and '40s. When it began to surface again, it did so in large part on the strength of various semantic subterfuges.

Mercy killing is a name that tells it as it is. The Austrian Christian scholar Hans Millendorfer defines euthanasia succinctly as "a method in which killing represents a solution." In increasingly post-Christian and politically correct America, however, killing is not a word we like to use. We have 1.5 million legal abortions annually, but we never speak of killing a developing fetus, much less of killing a baby. It is very hard to popularize a concept that includes the word killing, even when it is joined to *mercy*. Better labels have had to be found: As Mary Poppins sings, "A spoonful of sugar makes the medicine go down." The sugar on euthanasia is largely semantic: The terms death with dignity and right to die have made it progressively easier to swallow.

Our age is one in which rights are foremost, responsibilities hindmost. If a thing can be labeled a right, then it is almost certain to be popular. An individual is postulated to have the right to die, a right that must be granted him by society through the "care" of his doctor. (Recent articles in the *Journal of the American Medical Association* and the *New England Journal of Medicine* have begun to speak of "physician-assisted suicide in the *care* [emphasis added] of the terminally ill.") It is a curious kind of right that guarantees to us something that not one of us can avoid by any means at our disposal. It is, rather, as though one defined a right to eat as being force-fed even when one is not yet hungry.

Another important semantic tool in the mercy killing movement is the concept of death with dignity. Dignity in death used to have a meaning associated with the root meaning of the Latin word *dignus*, "worthy." Nathan Hale (hanged by a British court for spying for the American rebels) died with dignity in the old sense, a fact recognized even by his executioners, who allowed him time to pronounce his famous last words, "I only regret that I have but one life to lose for my country."

Death with dignity has come to mean something else again. Francis Schaeffer said most modern men and women are living only for "personal peace and affluence." When the ability to enjoy those things is being taken away, the cry goes up for "the release of life devoid of value," the slogan coined by the two theorists of the German euthanasia movement, Karl Binding and Alfred Hoche, in their 1920 publication bearing those words in its title. Unfortunately, the concepts "release of life" and "life devoid of value" are a bit too negative to go down well in modern America. They seem to be taking away rather than giving (which of course they are, but no one wants to look at it that way). And so *death with dignity* has been coined. We all want our rights and so might be expected to campaign even for the right to die, but *die*, standing all alone, remains an unpleasant word. Therefore one must die with dignity. The procedure envisioned by the euthanasia movement is similar to that used in putting an old dog or other beloved pet "to sleep," again a euphemism to cover an unpleasant reality: killing.

A dog or a cat has nothing to which to look forward when its bodily life is at an end, and thus it makes much sense—it is indeed a form of mercy—to speed that end by mercy killing. But human life—if the Bible is true, and indeed it is—has a different *telos*, a different goal and destination. Therefore it does not make sense to deal with humans, as life ebbs away, in the manner that · is appropriate for dogs and cats—and call it dignity.

The Hippocratic tradition pledges physicians to do all they can to heal. Curiously, for our modern sensibility, the oath says nothing about that modern desire that opens the door for mercy killing, namely, to relieve or end suffering. Modern physicians, despite the incredible advances in the healing arts, are finite human beings, just as Hippocrates was, and there will come a time for each of them—and for each of us—when their art and their artifices are all at an end. Then they must allow nature to take its course. To call this recognition of human finiteness, this graceful yielding to the necessity imposed upon each of us by the fall, passive euthanasia is to confuse fundamentally different things—killing and allowing to die—and to prepare the public to accept the still more "merciful" form, "active" euthanasia, or as Millendorfer put it, the "method in which killing represents a solution."

Death with dignity normally is not thought to be secured simply by allowing to die: It must be imposed, even enforced, by imposing that strange "right" to die; in other words, by mercy killing. Do we not like the word killing? Unless it is just the sound we do not like, we dare not swallow the surrogates right to die and death with dignity. If it is the thing in itself that we do not like, namely the killing of patients by their health-care professionals, we must relentlessly expose the sugary words intended to help the "medicine," that deadly draft, go down. If we love mercy, as God in his Word commands (Micah 6:8), we must shun euthanasia, for in the words of one honest physician, "Mercy killing kills mercy."

# The Right Questions

*Ken Myers*

Whenever it becomes possible to do what was previously unthinkable, one must exercise new moral muscles. A college student living away from home for the first time suddenly has choices about how to spend time, money, and self that were practically unavailable while living under the roof of wise and watchful parents. More important, if the student has not developed, by the grace of God, the sort of character that will enable him to live in a manner consistent with his convictions, all of his efforts at moral reasoning are likely to come to naught.

Modern technology, social order, and ideologies are not arrayed to create totally new contexts for moral decision-making. The wisdom of past generations sometimes seems to fail us when issues such as *in vitro* fertilization or the removal of life-support systems are before us. The pressures of modern technology and the philosophical tendencies of utilitarianism, pragmatism, and relativism influence the way we and our contemporaries answer questions relating to medical ethics.

27

What is not as well understood is the way modern experience shapes the way we *ask* questions, or encourages us to ask certain questions and to ignore others. With the modern dominance of science as a way of perceiving reality, religious or spiritual questions are considered at best private and sectarian, at worst superstitious nonsense.

But the scientific method also insists that natural phenomena be understood in isolation from the broader context in which they normally are found. Sociologist Brigitte Berger has noted that this principle has been transferred to our understanding of social realities. This makes it possible (and likely) that modern feminism will understand what it means to be a woman "in isolation from the wider structures of personal and social life, including those of the family." Thus arguments are made about a woman's right to abortion, not a mother's right to abortion. The woman is taken as an individualistic, atomistic entity, not as a person in a fabric of duties and responsibilities as well as rights.

The debate between prolife and proabortion forces on the personhood of the fetus may suffer from the same problem. Is the fetus a person? may be the wrong question, although it is the sort of question that scientific prejudices might elicit. Is that fetus your son or daughter? might be a better way of asking the question. Ethicist Stanley Hauerwas has written an essay titled "My Uncle Charlie Isn't Much of a Person, but He's Still My Uncle Charlie," which raises the same sort of question with regard to euthanasia. In other words, what is the most morally significant matter in medical ethical decisions: the category of personhood or the demands of kinship? Hauerwas believes Christians should not accept the terms of debate as defined by secular society. As biblical people, kinship is a powerful force. Our identity before God as creatures and as the elect is defined more in terms of a kinship than in abstract, ontological categories. This is not to dismiss such categories, only to suggest that they aren't the only morally compelling categories.

Another way modern society has influenced how ethical questions are raised is with its preoccupation with freedom. The question, Should people be allowed to do such-and-such? tends to eclipse questions such as, Is it right for anyone to do such-and-such? and, Is it prudent for a lot of people to do such-and-such? Christians usually are quick to recognize the moral relativism or pragmatism that ignores questions of right and wrong. We have lost the conviction of most earlier generations of believers that some things may be morally permissible but may be imprudent. The question, Is

*In debates about policies as well as in personal decisions that deal with medical ethics, Christians need to be increasingly alert to the issues needing answers and ably prepared to ask better questions.*

this a good thing to do? not only implies the question, Do I have a right to do such a thing? but, Is this the best thing to do? Believers are not called to pursue minimal morality but to pursue the greater good. Taken in isolation, a particular course of action may not be intrinsically sinful. But it may add momentum to dangerous and sinful tendencies in my own life, in the lives of my family members, or in my community.

Finally, our society is increasingly obsessed with self-fulfillment. Philip Rieff has noted that premodern cultures always functioned as mechanisms of restraint. In theological terms, cultures were means of common grace, keeping people from doing anything their depraved hearts wanted. But since the self-analytic and therapeutic mind-set has become established in the West, culture is now understood as having the duty to become a mechanism of liberation. Cultures should encourage and allow people to do anything they want because, according to the therapeutic mythology, self-fulfillment is the highest good in human experience.

In this setting, medical ethics often sees its task as determining what procedures, practices, and policies will promote self-fulfillment. So if a fetus or an elderly person is judged to be incapable of living a fulfilled life, that life becomes virtually worthless.

It is hard to get the right answers if the questions are wrong. In debates about policies as well as in personal decisions that deal with medical ethics, Christians need to be increasingly alert to the issues needing answers and ably prepared to ask better questions. Better questions don't always lead to easier answers or to answers that are easier to abide by. But like all generations of God's people striving toward obedience, we live in difficult times.

# Just Do Right

## George Grant

Knowing what is right is not nearly so difficult as doing what is right. Orthodoxy is a far simpler matter than orthopraxy.

Nowhere is that more evident than in the heart-wrenching issues of biomedical ethics. These days, Himalayan slogans naturally seem to accompany the fierce debate over what individuals and their physicians should and should not do. When it comes to the rhetorical tug-of-war over mercy, justice, and the sanctity of human life, we tend to throw battle cries and shibboleths as loosely as small change. Carried away by the emotional hurricanes of the moment, it is all too easy for us to forget that life-and-death decisions are agonizingly complex and require more than our unswerving dogma. They require our unswerving valor as well.

The world makes a pretense of easy answers. Abortion masquerades as an easy remedy for a difficult dilemma. Euthanasia, living will legislation, assisted suicide, and removal of nutrition and hydration all pose as easy solutions to intractable problems. Of course, we know they aren't. But then neither are the alternatives. Though there certainly are *right* answers, there are no *easy* answers. To pretend otherwise—even in the heat of battle—may paralyze the moral resolve of men and women in times of crisis.

> *The bottom line for us is that we simply cannot expect to preserve the biblical standard of the sanctity of human life in this fallen world if our message is merely propositional and solely negative.*

The import of this is evident throughout the Scriptures. Paul, for instance, not only preached the whats and whys of truth but the hows as well. He affirmed that knowing what was right had to be accompanied by the bravery to do it. Thus, following a string of dogmatic admonitions, he wrote: "Be on your guard, stand firm in the faith, be men of courage, be strong. Do everything in love" (1 Cor. 16:13–14).

Paul exhorted the Corinthians to recognize that choosing the right way requires real resistance to the prevailing wisdom of the world. And that is hard. There are no ifs, ands, or buts about it.

The bottom line for us is that we simply cannot expect to preserve the biblical standard of the sanctity of human life in this fallen world if our message is merely propositional and solely negative. Our challenge is not simply to teach *that* people should "just say no," but *how* to muster the courage to "just do right."

# But Lord, My Lawyer Said It Would Be Okay

*Kenneth L. Connor*

We live in an age of rapid change. The Greek philosopher Heraclitus observed, "All is flux, nothing stays still. Nothing endures but change." Rarely, however, has the rate of change proceeded at the pace it does today—especially in the areas of science and technology. And nowhere is change more apparent than in the fields of biology, medicine, and engineering. Rapid advancements in these fields have given rise to a new field, biomedical engineering. We are in the midst of a veritable biological revolution. Biological knowledge is doubling every five years; in the field of genetics, every two years.

The brave new worlds opened up by science and technology contain within them the seeds of hope and destruction. Advances in these fields have produced "miracle" cures that just a few years ago were unimaginable. But technology is a two-edged sword. The technology that is a blessing for some can, at the same time, be a curse for others. Fetal tissue transplants offer the hope of an enhanced quality of life for those suffering from Parkinson's disease, diabetes, and old age, but the improvements come at the expense of the lives of the unborn babies from whom the tissue is "harvested." *In vitro* fertilization offers the hope of children for infertile couples, but parenthood comes at the cost of the lives of the embryos who are discarded during the process. In utero screening for birth defects enables the early detection of genetic anomalies in children, but that knowledge often results in the destruction of the children who are deemed defective.

The application we make of our new technologies can give rise to profound legal and ethical dilemmas. Because of the dark side of technology, the question, Can I? in the technical sense often must be followed by the question, May I? in the legal sense. Far too often, however, the question that goes unasked is, Should I? Many well-meaning but naive people often assume that if something is legal it must be okay. That assumption is no longer valid, especially in the area of bioethical decision-making. Those who look only to the law for guidance in making sound bioethical decisions will be poorly served. The law is seldom an adequate ethical guide in the biomedical field. Here's why: Law follows rather than leads, it is inherently political, and it does not rest on transcendent values.

Advances in the biomedical arena are occurring so rapidly that they often occur in a legal vacuum. Frequently, there simply is no law that governs decision-making in a given area of biomedicine. The reason is that the fields of biology, medicine, and the law move at vastly different paces. Changes in the law, by design, occur at a ponderously slow pace. Delay is the hallmark of change in the law. Not so with science and technology. Thanks to the "magic" of silicone chips and other state-of-the-art technologies, changes are occurring so rapidly in scientific fields that by the time the law is applied to a given area, it is often out of date because technology has moved the field light years ahead. Decision-making in the biomedical field, thus, often occurs in uncharted legal waters. In a legal vacuum, that which is not prohibited is permitted. Merely because something is permitted, however, doesn't mean it is right.

Law is usually made in a highly charged political environment. Anyone who has been involved in the legislative process knows that the merits are often irrelevant to the outcome of a proposed law. Money, special interests, partisan politics, procedural high jinks, and political clout often drive the political process. Political expedience frequently prevails over principled decision-making. Because of this,

> *There was a period in American history when the civil law in America was rooted in the transcendent values found in Scripture.*

the law is seldom an adequate standard by which to gauge ethical decision-making in the biomedical field.

Legal rights are generally equated with freedoms. People tend to think of a legal right as the freedom to do or say or believe something without interference by the state or others. A legal "wrong" is viewed simply as an unauthorized encroachment on someone's legal rights. The legal right, in and of itself, is thus viewed as the standard by which a legal wrong is judged. There is no resort to a transcendent standard. Under the law, it is deemed wrong to violate one's legal rights.

In the arena of ethics, right and wrong are judged by a transcendent standard. Something is viewed as morally right or wrong based on whether it comports to a "higher" law. That higher law may be deemed the law of nature or of nature's God, but it is deemed to be, in all events, something that is greater than and other than the right itself.

There was a period in American history when the civil law in America was rooted in the transcendent values found in Scripture. It is precisely for this reason that Abraham Lincoln, arguing against the institution of slavery, maintained that "[no]body has a right to do wrong." His point very simply was that one should not have a legal right to do that which is morally wrong. Lincoln's argument would carry little weight in America today. In our "enlightened" secularized society, the linkage between legal rights and moral rights has been broken. Legal rights are seen simply as those rights that are conferred or recognized by the government. Morals and ultimate values may be deemed to have a place, but only outside the legal arena. Nowhere is this better illustrated than in the area of abortion. The "right" to abort a child results from the Supreme Court's decision to give primacy to so-called rights of privacy and personal autonomy. Because of the weight given by the Court to the interests an individual has in personal autonomy and privacy, a woman's right of privacy was deemed by the Court to outweigh any claim her unborn child had to a right to life. Nowhere in its decision did the Court address the morality of a mother killing her unborn child.

Scripture does not place much weight on interests such as privacy or personal autonomy. It teaches that everything we do occurs under the watchful eye of an omniscient, omnipotent God to whom we are accountable. Further, the Scriptures recognize the transcendent worth, value, and dignity of all individuals, including children. Children are regarded by Scripture as blessings for which we are to be thankful, not burdens that are to be discarded. A careful examination of Scripture on subjects relating to the sanctity of life, marriage, and the family (all of which are implicated in many biomedical decisions) yields numerous conflicts with our current civil law. Because of recent changes in the foundations of American law, Christians will do well to look to the law of God, as well as to the law of the land, when seeking guidance in making sound bioethical decisions.

The psalmist declared, "The [law] of the LORD [not the law of man] is sure, making wise the simple" (Ps. 19:7 KJV). Rarely are there decisions that call for greater wisdom than the life-and-death judgments that are involved in biomedical ethics. May God grant us the wisdom to discern not only that which is legal but also that which is right.

# Utilitarianism and the Moral Life

## J. P. Moreland

The goal of normative ethics is to develop a comprehensive, coherent system of morality that answers difficult questions. For advocates of biblical Christianity, whatever system we embrace should square with our considered, commonsense moral intuitions derived from natural law, and it should be consistent with, shed light upon, and help extend the morality contained in Scripture.

Currently, there are three competing normative systems. *Virtue ethics* does not focus primarily on moral rules (e.g., "don't steal") or moral actions but on describing the good person or community and the features present in a virtuous character. *Deontological ethics* (from *deon*, meaning "binding duty") focuses on moral rules and actions and emphasizes duty done for duty's sake. Certain moral rules are intrinsically correct and should be followed simply because they are right.

Virtue and deontological ethics are easily harmonized. But that is not the case with a third normative theory: *utilitarianism.*

Utilitarianism (also called consequentialism) is a moral theory developed and refined in the modern world by Jeremy Bentham (1748–1832) and John Stuart Mill (1806–73). It can be defined as follows: An action or moral rule is right if and only if it maximizes the amount of nonmoral good produced in the consequences that result from doing that act or following that rule compared with other acts or rules open to the agent.

By focusing on three features of utilitarianism, we can clarify this definition.

*1. Utilitarian theories of value.* What is a nonmoral good? Utilitarians deny there are any more actions or rules that are intrinsically right or wrong. But they do believe in objective values that are nonmoral.

*Hedonistic* utilitarians say that the only intrinsic good is pleasure and the avoidance of pain. Quantitative hedonists (Bentham) say the amount of pleasure and pain is the only thing that matters. In deciding between two courses of action, I should do the one that produces the greatest amount of pleasure and the least amount of pain. Qualitative hedonists (Mill) say pleasure is the only intrinsic good, but the type of pleasure is what is important, not the amount. They would rank pleasures that come from reading, art, and friendship as more valuable than those that come from, say, a full stomach.

*Pluralistic* utilitarians say a number of things have intrinsic, nonmoral value, such as pleasure, friendship, health, knowledge, freedom, peace, and security. For pluralists, it is not just the pleasure that comes from friendship that has value but also friendship itself.

Currently, the most popular utilitarian view of value is *subjective preference* utilitarianism. This position says it is presumptuous and impossible to specify things that have intrinsic nonmoral worth. So intrinsic value ought to be defined as that which each individual wants, provided it does not harm others. Unfortunately, this view collapses into moral relativism.

*2. Utilitarians and maximizing utility.* Utilitarians use the term *utility* to stand for whatever good they are seeking to produce as consequences of a moral action (e.g., "pleasure" for the hedonist, "satisfaction of subjective preference" for others). They see morality in a means-to ends way. The sole value of a moral action or rule is the utility of its consequences. Moral action should maximize utility. This can be interpreted in different ways, but many utilitarians embrace the following: The correct moral action or rule is the one that produces the greatest amount of utility for the greatest number of people.

> *In balancing positive and negative utilities, and excluding from the equation the objective sacredness of all human life, utilitarianism arrives at morally repugnant decisions.*

*3. Two forms: act utilitarianism, rule utilitarianism.* According to act utilitarianism, an act is right only if no other act available maximizes utility more than the act in question. Here, each new moral situation is evaluated on its own, and moral rules like "don't steal" or "don't break promises" are secondary. Rule utilitarianism says correct moral actions are done in keeping with correct moral rules. However, no moral rule is intrinsically right or wrong. Rather, a correct moral rule is one that would maximize utility if most people followed it instead of an alternative rule. Here, alternative rules (e.g., "don't lie" versus "don't lie unless doing so would enhance friendship") are compared for their consequences, not specific actions.

Several objections show the inadequacy of utilitarianism as a normative moral theory.

First, utilitarianism can justify actions that are clearly immoral. Consider the case of a severely deformed fetus. The child is certain to live a brief, albeit painless life. He or she will make no contribution to society. Society, however, will bear great expense. Doctors and other caregivers will invest time, emotion, and effort in adding mere hours to the baby's life. The parents will know and love the child only long enough to be heartbroken at the inevitable loss. An abortion would negate all those "utility" losses. Therefore, the child should be aborted. In balancing positive and negative utilities, and excluding from the equation the objective sacredness of all human life, utilitarianism arrives at morally repugnant decisions. Deontological and virtue ethics, on the other hand, would steer us clear of what is easier to what is right.

Second, in a similar way, utilitarianism denies the existence of acts of moral heroism that are not morally obligatory but are still praiseworthy. Examples would be giving 75 percent of your income to the poor or throwing yourself on a bomb to save a stranger. Consider the bomb example. You have two choices—throwing yourself on the bomb or not doing so. Each choice would have consequences, and according to utilitarianism, you are morally obligated to do one or the other depending on which option maximizes utility. Thus, there is no room for acts that go beyond the call of morality.

Third, utilitarianism has an inadequate view of human rights and dignity. If enslaving a minority of people, say by a lottery, would produce the greatest good for the greatest number, or if conceiving children only to harvest their parts would do the same, then these could be justified in a utilitarian scheme. But they would violate individual rights and treat people as a means to an end, not as creatures with intrinsic dignity. If abortion, active euthanasia, physician-assisted suicide, and the like maximize utility, then they are morally obligatory for the utilitarian. But any system that makes abortion and suicide morally obligatory is surely flawed.

Finally, utilitarianism has an inadequate view of motives and character. Utilitarianism implies that the only reason we should praise good motives instead of bad ones, or seek good character instead of bad character, is because such acts would maximize utility. But this has the cart before the horse. We should praise good motives or character and blame bad ones because they are intrinsically good or bad, not because praising and blaming produce good consequences.

It should be clear that utilitarianism is an inadequate moral theory. Unfortunately, ours is a pragmatic culture and utilitarianism is on the rise. But for those of us who follow Christ, a combination of virtue and deontological ethics is a more adequate view of common sense morality found in natural law and of the moral vision contained in the Bible. As such, it is the better view on which to base our approach to the difficult issues raised in today's biomedical ethics.

# An Unchanging Standard

*R. C. Sproul*

Recently, the Vatican announced the release of a new catechism, a massive work years in the making. I am eagerly awaiting its translation into English. My interest is not dominated by a new theological dictum but by what the document will say on the field of biomedical ethics.

Roman Catholic moral theology has been one of the church's strong suits. Catholic scholars have placed a premium on the careful exploration of ethical issues. Though I frequently differ with Rome in its moral theology, I have an abiding respect for the care of its work. Rome refuses to be held hostage by societal shifts in customs or mores. It doesn't decide moral issues by referendum.

In the arena of biomedical ethics, we face a unique problem. In the general field of ethics, we have the advantage of two thousand years of careful research, debate, and insight into complex and weighty problems. With biomedical ethical issues that confront us, however, we do not have the benefit of such long-term investigation. The use of life-support systems, *in vitro* fertilization, and other technologies has introduced new dilemmas and poses new ethical questions.

To address these questions, we have the advantage of manifold basic principles. It is the application of such principles to complex new problems that is difficult.

These problems are not restricted to abstract theoretical questions. They are issues that touch heavily on life itself. With increasing regularity pastors are called to assist in decision-making crises that involve the use of life-support systems. The question of when to "pull the plug" touches life issues so poignantly that to avoid paralyzing guilt problems, the pastor, along with the attending physician, is asked to play God.

But no pastor is God. We look to our pastor to give us the voice of God. We want God's guidance in these ethical dilemmas. The Supreme Court is not an adequate substitute for the person who is more concerned to discern and to carry out what is right rather than simply what is legal.

> *The great conflict between relativism and absolutism is the conflict between the will of the creature and the will of the Creator.*

To solve such dilemmas, we need clear and normative principles. Principles exist in the abstract. Decisions must be made in concrete life situations, although those situations do not dictate the decision. We do not have the luxury of making no decision. To make no decision is to make a decision.

What we are after in biomedical ethics are clear and certain principles that are not arbitrary. We need principles that are absolute and normative. The legal code of society can never provide an absolute norm. In societies where laws are enacted according to popular will, the result is conflicting and contradictory laws. In the United States abortion is legal. In Ireland abortion is illegal. Does this mean that it is ethically right to abort American babies but wrong to abort Irish babies? Or to put it another way, was it ethically wrong to have an abortion before *Roe v. Wade* but ethically proper after *Roe v. Wade?* If legal rights are an absolute norm, we would say yes.

The ultimate standard of right and wrong is the character of God as revealed in his law. God's law must be applied in given situations, but the good should never be dictated by the situation. The situation is subordinate to the principle, not the principle to the situation.

"New morality" follows the situation ethics set forth popularly by Joseph Fletcher. Fletcher summarized his view of ethics by saying, "We must always do what love requires in the situation."

This maxim, if it stood alone, would be sound. We are always responsible to do what love demands in a situation. Love is the linchpin of the law of God. The problem remains how to know what love requires in a given situation. God's law reveals what God's love requires.

When Paul speaks of the ethics of love, he says, "And live a life of love, just as Christ loved us . . ." (Eph. 5:2). But the apostle does not stop with an ambiguous appeal to love. In the next breath he says, "But among you there must not be even a hint of sexual immorality, or any kind of impurity, or of greed, because these are improper for God's holy people" (Eph. 5:3).

Here the law of God defines what is consistent with love. Appeals to love are frequently used to excuse sin. The oldest ploy in the world for sexual seduction is, "If you love me, you will." Yet Paul declares, "If you love God, you won't. Ever."

Most ethical decisions we face involve the application of more than one principle. Balancing the myriad principles of the law of God requires wisdom. To face the new questions posed in the field of biomedical ethics, we must grasp the relevant principles that apply.

Professor John Frame of Westminster Seminary West has contributed greatly to the discussion with his book *Biomedical Ethics*. Likewise, John Jefferson Davis has also helped with his work *Evangelical Ethics*. We must continue to study the questions in light of biblical principles as we seek to live under the authority of God and for his glory. His principles are not subject to the shifting sands of cultural or legal relativism.

God's law is law. It requires a response of obedience for which we are held accountable. The last judgment prophesied by the New Testament refers to a final and absolute tribunal from which there is no court of appeal. This tribunal is a cosmic supreme court. Lawlessness and disobedience will be punished according to justice. Obedience will result in the distribution of rewards.

In the scenario of final judgment, the folly of relativism will be fully exposed. The wisdom and excellence of divine law will be manifest.

The absolute law of God reveals the absolute glory and righteousness of God. It reflects God's own character, his own righteousness. It also expresses the authority of God by which he rules by divine right. As the author of creation, God has the authority to command from his creatures what he deems right.

The great conflict between relativism and absolutism is the conflict between the will of the creature and the will of the Creator. In relativism the individual is the final authority for behavior. It is the syndrome described by Scripture as each person doing "what is right in his own eyes." This conflict is as old as human experience after the fall.

The law of God transcends individual preferences. It provides an objective norm, a norm that governs everybody's behavior. The norm is revealed, giving each of us the opportunity and the responsibility to know what righteousness requires of us in life situations. If we fail to apply God's standard, we are left with no excuse.

# Part 2

# Manipulating the Body

I was only seven when I was sidelined for six months with a broken leg. I remember reading a lot, but also watching too much television. During the days the Watergate trials droned on and on. One night, however, I came across a new show that caught my attention. As the opening credits ran, a solemn voice intoned, "We have the technology, we can rebuild him." The show was about a government test pilot who became a sort of superhero. In a terrible crash, he lost both legs, an arm, and an eye. They were replaced with machines, bionic machines. The price tag? Six million dollars. The $6 million man could run sixty miles an hour without tiring, lift automobiles with one arm, and see for miles.

It was enough to leave any seven-year-old boy bug-eyed. Television did not so destroy my imagination that I couldn't envision myself performing such feats. More than two decades later, little is left to the imagination. Technology has radically changed the way we view our bodies. We have the technology, we can rebuild ourselves.

The price tag, however, is well beyond a mere $6 million. As a culture we have sold our souls to rebuild our bodies. Beyond the obvious costs of aborted fetuses used to harvest ova, or siblings conceived for bone marrow transplants, is the cost of our selves. The miracles of medical technologies have led us to see our bodies not as miracles but as tools. Technology has led us to accept Plato's old lie that we are mere ghosts in machines. Too much of this technology has created not superheroes but an army of Dr. Frankensteins.

We are not souls in bodies but souls and bodies. From the creation of Adam to the resurrection of the Second Adam, the Scriptures tell us that our bodies are not means to ends but ends themselves. Our salvation is not merely the salvation of souls. We are saved body and soul. Christ died, in part, to save our bodies. When he comes again he will take us with him, body and soul. It is important to consider that truth as we strive to resolve increasingly complex dilemmas in health care and life-and-death issues.

Living *coram Deo*, before the face of God, always means gratitude. We must be thankful for both the creation and redemption of our souls. We also must give thanks for the creation and redemption of our bodies.

# You Shall Not Be Gods

## R. C. Sproul

"You shall be like gods" (KJV). This was the original temptation, the archetypal seduction aimed at our first parents by the serpent. Created as vice-regents with dominion over the earth, Adam and Eve wanted more. They reached for autonomy, stretching greedy arms toward the throne of God, only to fall headlong into the abyss of evil. Expulsion from Eden was their fate. They could not go back. Paradise was lost. An angel with a flaming sword stood guard at the gateway to the garden. This is the first reference in Scripture to a weapon of any sort. Before God gave the "power of the sword" to men, he gave it to the angel to patrol and guard the border west of Nod.

With the fall came a rapid expansion of sin. One son of Adam and Eve murdered his brother, introducing fratricide to human history. This violence was followed by Lamech, who celebrated warfare in his famous "sword song" (Gen. 4:23–24). Man, originally given dominion and called to dress, till, and replenish the earth, used his nascent technology to turn the tools of farming into implements of war. The plowshare became a sword, and the call to subdue the earth was distorted into a conspiracy to conquer one's brother. The means of production became the means of destruction, and human technology and scientific discovery were used not to honor God but to assault him, by attacking his creation and his image-bearers.

Then God said no to the expansion of corruption and brought the flood, a storm of judgment upon the earth, a deluge to clean the planet.

After the flood, Noah and his family began to repopulate the earth. Noah's descendants became hunters (Nimrod) and builders. A new technology emerged to provide stabler and more suitable shelter. Brick and mortar became the means by which whole cities could be built: "'Come let's make bricks and bake them thoroughly.' They used brick instead of stone, and tar for mortar. Then they said, 'Come, let us build ourselves a city, with a tower that reaches to the heavens, so that we may make a name for ourselves . . .'" (Gen. 11:3–4).

> *We still grasp for autonomy, refusing to have God rule over us.*

Immediately after the flood, Noah erected an altar, a structure upon which to offer the sacrifice of praise and worship. The building project at Babel was something else. Again it was a reach of pretended autonomy, a stretch for heaven, an attempt to rip God down from his throne that man might make for *himself* a name. The result of this effort, this primitive scientific undertaking, was chaos. The language of man was confused, and communication gave way to babbling.

This pattern has not changed. The greater the technology, the greater the chaos. The more sophisticated the tools, the more sophisticated the violence. The twentieth century is the age of high technology. The technological advances of our age have eclipsed all previous generations. The most peaceful century in human history was the first century. The second most peaceful century was the nineteenth. That century evoked an unprecedented spirit of human optimism. The Enlightenment concluded that man no longer needs the God-hypothesis to explain his origins and purpose. An optimistic humanism was born that promised a coming utopia. Education, science, and technology would produce the acme of evolutionary development. Peace would prevail, and poverty, disease, crime, and war would be banished by the modern techniques of government, economics, and education.

World War I temporarily burst the bubble until it was decreed the war to end all wars. Somebody forgot to tell that to the sons of Lamech: Mussolini, Tojo, Stalin, Mao, and the corporal from Bavaria. The twentieth century brought a new horror to world history, the phenomenon of global war. The new warfare engaged alliances from east and west in wars numbered by roman numerals and punctuated by a mushroom cloud.

We cannot blame this on technology. It is not the instruments that are culpable; it is the users of the instruments. The same scalpel that is used to save a life in surgery is now used to hack into pieces millions of unborn babies. The same atomic energy that supplies power for living is harnessed for weapons of incalculable destruction.

The technological explosion proliferates in geometric proportion. Yet the human spirit of corruption remains. We are still trying to be as God. We still grasp for autonomy, refusing to have God rule over us. We now reach beyond the heights of an ancient ziggurat. We walk on the moon and call it a real step forward for mankind.

We are indeed "enlightened." No longer do students carry switchblades to school. They carry guns. Gangsters don't use tommy guns. Machine Gun Kelly has become obsolete in the face of assault weapons and rocket launchers. The battering ram has yielded to the ICBM. Our cities are armed fortresses, and we need more brick and mortar for prisons. We are still confused. Our politicians babble to us daily on the magic technology of television. And still everyone does what is right in his own eyes.

Marx believed that whoever controls the means of production (tools) controls the world. The race for technological supremacy is the race for dominion. Autonomy is the objective. But there is no technology sophisticated enough to fulfill the serpent's seductive promise. We are not gods. We shall not be gods. We cannot be gods. Only God can be God. Only God can be supreme. The issue in Eden is the issue today: Who will have dominion over man and man's technology? Our margin of error shrinks each day. Now we have the technology and techniques not to destroy God but to destroy ourselves. It is technological madness.

# The Promise
# of Prozac and Silicone

*Randy Crenshaw*

Broken promises litter the landscape of the American dream.

Our physicians and scientists told us they had the secrets to help us find satisfaction. They promised to make us beautiful and made millionaires of our plastic surgeons; they claimed changing our brain chemistry would make us content and propelled Prozac into fourth place on the best-seller list; they purported that eating right and exercising would bring us peace of mind and long life, and spawned a burgeoning business of health spas and weight loss clinics.

This is the "morning after" for American medicine. We have awakened to find that promises made in the heat of commercial passion look much less certain in the blinding light of day. The dreams of thousands of women exploded when their silicone breast implants ruptured. The thick, slippery gel oozed out into the surrounding tissue, and many developed vague symptoms of systemic sickness.

Expensive new drugs for depression work only half of the time. Placebos (sugar tablets) work in 20 to 30 percent of the cases. No one can say for sure how valid the research is because most depression gets better without treatment of any sort.

Doctors have been telling us for years that taking vitamins is a waste of time. Recent evidence reveals vitamin gulping may be positively harmful. The long-term success rate of diets and weight loss programs is dismally low, probably no better than 10 percent.

One hundred and fifty years ago, Americans ignored the promises made by the medical profession. Physicians were not esteemed by the public. Then technological improvements, such as X rays and microscopes, changed our view of the medicine men. Since scientists could "see" things mere mortals could not, we ascribed powers to them and gave them cultural authority.

The demand for medical care gets stronger every year. Yet the medical profession itself is raising serious questions about the value of those services. Yes, we are living a little longer; most of the gain, though, has occurred at the beginning of life. In 1900 the life expectancy of a seven-year-old was sixty-four years. Today it is seventy-two—hardly a quantum leap. Psalm 90:10 holds true: our years are seventy or eighty, and manipulation of our bodies will not increase them.

*Broken promises litter the landscape of the American dream.*

Some may say modern medical techniques have made the quality of life so much better, even if the span of life is not much longer. I suppose that depends on one's definition of quality. Former Secretary of Education William J. Bennett, in *The De-Valuing of America*, highlighted the decline of American culture over the last thirty years. He discovered "there has been a 560 percent increase in violent crime; a 410 percent increase in illegitimate births; a quadrupling of divorce rates; a tripling of the percentage of children living in single parent homes; more than a 200 percent increase in the teenage suicide rate; and a drop of almost 80 points in SAT scores." This is improvement?

Something is wrong here. We have been deceived. Plastic surgery, steroids, psychotropic drugs, health foods, fitness clubs, and assorted techniques have not made us healthier. They have only made us poorer. We have forgotten that God's wisdom outshines that of man.

In 1 Timothy 4:8, Paul addresses the issue of exercise, saying, "Physical training is of some value, but godliness has value for all things, holding promise for both the present life and the life to come."

Psalm 42:5–6 reveals an ancient prescription for depression: "Why are you downcast, O my soul? Why so disturbed within me? Put your hope in God, for I will yet praise him, my Savior and my God."

Peter shares the secret of personal beauty when he says, "Your beauty should not come from outward adornment, such as braided hair and the wearing of gold jewelry and fine clothes. Instead, it should be that of your inner self, the unfading beauty of a gentle and quiet spirit, which is of great worth in God's sight" (1 Peter 3:3–4).

I'm not saying drugs are never useful in treating depression. Many people, including Christians, have been helped by their judicious, temporary use. Not every swoon of the spirit, however, calls for popping a Prozac. Actually, if you are not sometimes intensely sad, living in a world estranged from God, you are mired deep in the mud of denial.

Neither am I suggesting Christians should despise beauty. On the contrary, under the influence of the Reformation, painters, musicians, and authors faithfully portrayed the beauty of the universe and glorified God, its Creator. God's instructions to the builders of the temple under Solomon's supervision likewise testify to his aesthetic nature.

And there is nothing wrong, per se, with exercising and making ourselves look good. We should want to take care of our bodies because they are temples of the Holy Spirit. The fault with most of our manipulations of the body lies in our motives. Succumbing to the spirit of the age, we are not content with what we have or who we are, and we are determined to change things.

To avoid falling into the world's trap, above all remember God made us. In our disappointment over how our lives are turning out, we should take consolation in knowing he loves us. He does not change us because we demand that he do so, and he is not obligated to explain why things are not the way we want them to be. He whispers to us to rest in the fact that one day he will bring everything to a righteous and joyous conclusion.

Meanwhile he has provided a way for us to be healthy—the way of the cross. The Scripture says we are "healed" by his wounds. When the Bible talks about health and healing, it most often uses the word *shalom*. We translate it peace, prosperity, satisfaction, or contentment—the very things we all long for. We find healthiness, contentment, and satisfaction by following Christ's example—denying ourselves the relief sin provides when life is hard.

The world says being healthy means having a low cholesterol level and clean arteries. The Bible says it means having a low level of self-centeredness and a clean heart. One comes through drugs and surgery, from those who have broken promises and given false hope. The other comes through repentance and faith in Jesus Christ, the God-man who keeps all his promises.

11

# Prenatal Techniques

*W. Andrew Hoffecker*

For thousands of years, the marriage bed, governed by God's moral law, represented how people carried out the command, "Be fruitful and multiply." But today's technology threatens to revolutionize how and under what conditions we procreate. Instead of conceiving a child by the traditional marital union, prenatal technologies offer a smorgasbord of options. Imagine an infant having as many as five "natural parents"—sperm donor, egg donor, surrogate mother, and two adults who actually raise the child. What prenatal technology makes this scenario possible?

Welcome to the age of eugenics (genetic engineering), in which people desire to improve the human race by controlling and manipulating genes. Eugenics isn't new. More than forty years ago, scientists discovered DNA, which one of the scientists dubbed "the secret of life." DNA provides a biological blueprint for living organisms. Manipulating this "secret of life" gave scientists the power to cross into an uncharted universe of conception morality.

Today, procedures which influence offspring by manipulating DNA are burgeoning. Their growth exposes ethical dilemmas, such as how much eugenics Christians should encourage—if any. For example, eugenics extremists believe they should prevent would-be parents with defective genes from producing children. Obviously, if abused, eugenics may fall headlong into a black hole which reduces God's blessing of procreation into selective human breeding. But do all eugenics, such as *in vitro* fertilization, gene splicing, and sperm banks, necessarily foreshadow the nightmare of test-tube baby farms prophesied by Huxley's *Brave New World*?

We ought to note that eugenics is a double-edged sword. Many couples thank God that prenatal tests indicate a genetic defect, thus warning them about the dangers of that pregnancy. On the other hand, in 1992 one genetic diagnostic procedure used to screen defects in several cases was believed responsible for actually causing birth defects. As in many scientific advances, ethical problems tend to arise when new procedures are used without guidance from transcendent moral law. Although some prenatal tests detect dangers in unborn babies, these procedures may also cause death. Who makes the decision?

*Imagine an infant having as many as five "natural parents" — sperm donor, egg donor, surrogate mother, and two adults who actually raise the child.*

Eugenic techniques encourage people to play God by tempting them to control the shaping of their progeny—from IQ to eye color.

Where better to shape your future child's destiny than in a sperm bank? There sperm is bought, stored, and sold. During the 1991 Persian Gulf War, before leaving for an uncertain future, some soldiers ensured if they did not return, their wives could still bear their children by "freezing assets" at local sperm banks. And infertile couples now can purchase sperm which will enable the wife to experience the joy of bearing her own child. Lest one think this a prenatal utopia, some social engineers are beginning to use these banks exclusively as a safety deposit for future "blue-chip babies." One notable sperm bank collects sperm only from Nobel prize-winning scientists. However, even the best laid plans of genetic engineers can run amok. In 1982 a scandal erupted when reporters revealed that two parents who purchased "elite" sperm found their product came not from geniuses but convicted felons.

Moral questions about eugenics go far beyond sperm banks. Recently much has been written about uniting sperm and eggs in a petri dish to produce embryos which later will be implanted in a woman's womb. Supporters believe this process, *in vitro* fertilization (IVF), is eugenics' solution to impotency, frigidity, childless single women, and myriad other conception problems. In contrast, critics fear IVF will usher in Bokanovsky's Process in *Brave New World*. Remember the Alpha and Beta test-tube babies? Scientists decanted children as Alphas and Betas to serve in superior positions while Gammas through Epsilons were bred to perform menial tasks. Today's taxpayers are less philosophical, but they watch IVF's dollar signs. Will high-tech baby production affect insurance rates if it's included under maternity coverage? Today IVF costs $7,000 to $11,000 per procedure, and in 1993 the bill for all services totaled more than $1 billion.

Like sperm banks, IVF unsheathes eugenics' moral double-edged sword. Eugenic procedures help infertile couples; however, before we say that IVF sounds too good to be bad, we remember the Alphas' and Betas' brave new world. Where do Christians find guidelines to petri-dish ethics?

Genesis tells us God ordained marriage so husband and wife would come together to procreate. If an infertile couple chose to implant another person's sperm and/or egg, would that resemble adultery? What happens to surplus or defective embryos—fetuses in the earliest stage of gestation—not implanted? How would destruction of those embryos differ from abortion? Will people use IVF to screen embryos that have defective genes (defined as anything from congenital diseases to wrong eye color)? In 1990 such questions led the Christian Medical and Dental Society (CMDS) to approve IVF—but only if sperm and egg are provided by husband and wife. The CMDS opposed experimenting with or discarding unused embryos. It also condemned the use of surrogate mothers.

Should we emulate the CMDS's courageous stand? Increasingly, danger signals flash. The moral dangers of back-to-the-future eugenics abound. A recent article discussed scientific experiments using the eggs from aborted mouse fetuses to impregnate another mouse. One editorial projected that before long, women may abort a female embryo so that later in life, at age fifty or sixty, they could be impregnated or use a surrogate mother to produce their own grandchildren. Will unchecked techniques tempt humans to kill so they can manipulate their own procreation?

Andrew Kimbrell reports in *The Human Body Shop* that more than fifty couples have produced babies to procure tissue for an existing child. Assuming current trends continue, one can make the poignant case that bizarre uses of genetic engineering will multiply. Some observers warn that future eugenics laboratories will resemble auto parts stores.

As we approach the twenty-first century, interpreting God's command to be fruitful and multiply becomes increasingly complicated. Although some herald DNA as the secret of life, it, like Eden's fruit, can easily tempt us to become as gods and make our own rules. Families and marriages are not value-neutral, nor is eugenics free from God's moral law. Will eugenics become another killing field? Or will we choose Scripture to steer our course for a healthier human race?

# The Human Body Shop

## Ken Myers

One critic of much of current biotechnological research is
Andrew Kimbrell, policy director of the Foundation on
Economic Trends in Washington, D.C., and author of *The
Human Body Shop: The Engineering and Marketing of Life*.
Kimbrell was interviewed for *Tabletalk* by columnist Ken Myers.

**Myers:** What are the most important policy issues that concern the engineering and marketing of life?

**Kimbrell:** What we're increasingly seeing is that as technology advances, more and more of the human body and
human body forms now are becoming economically valuable,
and are becoming subject to manipulation and marketing. Obviously when transfusions came around, blood became valuable;
it's currently being sold. The same with organ transplants and
organs. Reproductive technology has made sperm, eggs, and
women's reproductive systems valuable, and now we've seen
each of those elements either for sale or, in the case of women's
reproductive elements, for rent. With the advent of genetic

69

engineering, we've got the marketing of all 100,000 or more human genes. And we have a major controversy going on right now about whether multinational companies can actually patent the 100,000 genes that make up the human genome. The patent office and most of those involved feel that that will happen. We've had dozens of applications for a variety of human genes, including human brain genes.

Consider the human cloning debate. Several months ago researchers announced what many of us knew for a long time, that they were actually cloning human beings, taking early-stage embryos and using a variety of techniques to make twins, and sometimes ten or twenty copies of the same embryo. These embryos can be valuable in the fertility industry, for couples who either can produce only a limited amount of embryos or can't produce embryos at all. These fertility clinics can provide them with "top quality" embryos.

The National Institute of Health has convened a panel to approve federal funding for the cloning of human embryos, the manipulation of human embryos, including the taking of human embryos at the early cell division, taking out four cells and putting in four cells of an animal, a process called cell fusion. We've done it with animals, but never with a human and an animal. They want to see what happens over the next two or three weeks to that embryo. We certainly have reached the stage where we can not only manipulate human and ani-mal genes but also we are approaching the stage where we can do about what we want with human embryos. It should be noted that a couple of years back, the Trademark Office of the United States said that you could patent an embryo. So what we have is a real possibility of an *in vitro* fertilization clinic finding a really nice line of boy and girl—

**Myers:** Designer embryos?

**Kimbrell:** Right. You get blond hair and blue eyes if that's what you want, cloning that line of embryos, keeping any number of them in the freezer. When a couple comes that cannot produce embryos of their own, or one that can but they don't like the characteristics they have, they could look through a catalog and choose embryo line A or B, which will have been patented by the IVF Clinic. This is not science fiction today but science fact—and legal fact in the U.S.

*If God is dead, Dostoyevsky observed, everything is permitted. Nowhere is that prophecy more evident than in current research in biotechnology.*

**Myers:** How would you characterize the most focused theological objection to this, from a Christian standpoint?

**Kimbrell:** Christians have always insisted that the human body is created in the image of God, giving extraordinary dignity and meaning to the body itself. It's terribly important in the Judeo-Christian tradition.

Over the last two or three centuries, we've seen a long-term transition from the body as sacred to the body as secular. Instead of the body being the image of God, we now see it as a biological machine, in essence no different from the other machines with which we work. A recent *New York Times* editorial said that life is special, human life even more so, but biological machines are still machines that can be cloned, engineered, and patented. A major geneticist has said that for three thousand years there was this concept that life was sacred, but not anymore. Genetic engineering allows us to understand that we are all biological machines.

We are in an ethical free fall with thinking about the body where we no longer have any taboos that come from our concept of the body as sacred. Instead we're seeing the body more as just another commodity in the marketplace, whose elements we can sell. The consequences are extremely profound.

**Myers:** Christians have not been very successful at staying alert to the new issues or at mounting a careful resistance to them. Why do you think that's the case?

**Kimbrell:** One of the problems is that so many extraordinary advances in the new biological technologies come at us one at a time. We hear of cloning of embryos, then we hear of the creation of animals with human genes, then surrogate motherhood, then fetal organs being used in transplants, and they all seem somewhat unconnected. We need to understand in all of this that there are two major lines of advances in the biotechnology revolution.

One is the increasing commercialization of the body. The body is becoming a commodity. It started with our blood and organs, now it's invaded our reproductive system, embryos and fetal life, and genes. As technologies advance, all of this has become a commodity. And it's a slippery slope where we now see the patenting of life-forms and the ownership of what is certainly our common heritage and our common gift: the genetic makeup of the human body.

The second, again, is technology-driven: our ability to engineer life-forms to suit our own purposes. Once again, you see a massive devolution of our concept of life from sacred to secular, to viewing the whole of the biological community as nothing more than many machines, systems, that we can manipulate for whatever purpose we want. I think that if you look down the line, first we started engineering microbes (plants, animals), and now the human body itself, because we are in this ethical free fall.

The solutions to this, fortunately, are not complicated. First, as a society, and I think the whole Christian community, we need to firmly state that whether it be blood, organs, fetal life, women's reproductive systems, or genes, these are not for sale. Our tradition does not allow us to do that. Christians must say to that that it does not comport to the idea of the body as *imago Dei*.

Second, the same is true of the genetic engineering of life. I think that changing the permanent genetic code of animals and human beings to suit our needs is the final insult to the Creator, saying that the animals, and our own bodies, as they have been given to us, can and should be altered to suit whatever economic purposes a particular company has. I think it's very important that we carefully monitor, and declare a moratorium on, any permanent genetic alterations of animals or humans until we have thoroughly gauged the ethics of this.

We may reach a time in the future when we can correctly use this genetic manipulation to cure some pernicious human diseases, but at this point, we simply don't have the wisdom, understanding, or sacred context which would allow us to safely become coauthors of human evolution.

# Can You Clone a Soul?

## Michael S. Beates

Never has a culture been so healthy in body but so sick in soul. We have the world's best health clubs and doctors who specialize in every part of the body. But we also have the world's highest demand for psychiatrists and counselors. We quickly and too easily dispose of marriages and relationships—at great emotional, mental, and spiritual cost—while keeping our bodies trim, fit, and tanned. People live longer, but they often do so in anguish and loneliness of soul. We have separated our bodies from our souls.

Scripture paints a different picture: man as a holistic being; the body and soul as a dynamic unity; the physical/material as inseparable from the metaphysical/spiritual. In his book *Concise Theology: A Guide to Historic Christian Beliefs*, Dr. J. I. Packer concurs, writing, "Each human being in this world consists of a material body animated by an immaterial personal self. Scripture calls this self a *soul* or *spirit*. The embodiment of the soul is integral to God's design for mankind. . . . At death the soul leaves the defunct body behind, but . . . the Christian hope is not for redemption *from* the body but redemption *of* the body. Though the exact composition of our future glorified bodies is presently unknown, we know there will be some sort of continuity with our present bodies" (74–75).

It seems to me that at the root of our cultural obsession to manipulate the body is a fear of losing the body. This is justifiable fear for people with unregenerate souls. When the soul is dead, life in the body *is* all that remains, and such people understandably hold to it with tenacity. Thus, we should not be surprised by the radical attempts emerging from medicine and science to maintain and extend life in the body at all costs to the soul and to other bodies.

Consider a couple of examples. First, cannibalistic manipulation of the body extends life by "harvesting" fetal brain tissue from aborted babies for use in the brains of people with Parkinson's disease. Since Bill Clinton removed the ban on fetal tissue research, this practice has surged forward full speed. One Colorado clinic is engaged in a study of the effectiveness of such tissue transplants. Several dozen people with Parkinson's will undergo surgery, having their skulls opened for the implantation of tissue. But to see if there is a psychosomatic element in this procedure, only half will receive fetal tissue transplants. Such testing, manipulating the body with no intention of corrective measure, further diminishes the credibility of those engaged in such research.

> *At the root of our cultural obsession to manipulate the body is a fear of losing the body.*

Second, technology recently has achieved the ability to clone human beings by imitating what happens in the formation of identical twins. Scientists split the cells of a two- to eight-cell human embryo, creating two embryos of identical genetic makeup. Conceivably this could be done multiple times. Speculating as to how such a technology could be used, Charles Colson has said, "The answer reads like science fiction. Parents could use *in vitro* fertilization, separate the cells, and select one for genetic testing. If the test revealed defects, the remaining embryos could be destroyed; if the test was normal, the embryos could be implanted in the mother's womb. Scientists have also suggested freezing the extra embryos for future use. For example, if the original child dies at an early age, a frozen twin [embryo] could be thawed out, and the parents could raise a clone identical to the child they lost. Or what if the original child needs an organ transplant? Just unfreeze a twin and use it for spare parts. The tissue would match perfectly."

> *Our value as people, our personhood, comes not from what we do but from what we are.*

But such manipulation of unborn, genetically complete, and unique humans devalues all human life. Many contend, though, that embryos have less value since they are not conscious, useful persons. Our usefulness in body should never be the criterion for judging our value. Our value as people, our personhood, comes not from what we do but from what we are. Dr. Seuss had it right in his children's book *Horton Hears a Who* when he wrote, "A person is a person no matter how small."

We do well to remember Paul's words in Philippians 1:20–26. He desired to leave his body to be with Christ, which would be far better. But for the sake of the gospel, Paul was willing to stay in this earthly tent for a while longer so Christ and his church might be built up.

Richard Baxter, a seventeenth-century Puritan, is another good example. Plagued by numerous chronic conditions throughout his life (before the advent of pain-relief medications), he began at age thirty a daily discipline of meditating for half an hour on the life hereafter. This exercise of soul strengthened him for service and devotion to the kingdom's work well into his seventies. His anticipation of glory energized him day by day through aches and pains that you and I can easily erase by manipulating our bodies with Tylenol or the like. How easily we substitute a temporary physical remedy for the more lasting spiritual benefit. As you or ones you love face such issues, remember our Lord's admonition, "What good will it be for a man if he gains the whole world, yet loses his soul?" (Matt. 16:26).

# Technology and the New Gnosticism

*Ken Myers*

Years ago the slogan used by DuPont was "Better things for better living through chemistry." Sometime in the '60s or '70s, the final prepositional phrase was dropped from the motto, presumably because the cultural affinity for things natural had jaundiced public opinion toward things chemical.

There is an assumption still at work in the shortened version of the slogan that one can advance on the ideal of the good life by improving one's material surroundings.

I'm writing this column on a fairly sophisticated computer. The air conditioner is droning in the background, eliminating some of the midsummer humidity, though obscuring some of the beauty of the music by William Byrd that is playing on the CD player. When I finish writing this piece, I will send it by fax (since I am, as usual, late in finishing it) to the good people at

Ligonier Ministries. They will use their computers and other technical wonders to place it in your hands, and, it is hoped, when you read it, you will gain some small bit of wisdom that will enable you to be a more thoughtful Christian. Your life might be made better. Technology (including some chemistry) thereby has fulfilled the mission of science envisioned by Francis Bacon: "For the relief of man's estate."

I am not antitechnology. But there is room to worry about how science and technology shape our lives. They are good gifts of God to sinful people, who are capable of discovering ways to misuse even the best gifts.

Some of the most awesome technology in our time is employed in the most urgent relief of man's estate, in biomedical applications. In one sense such procedures and devices might be seen as the best of the gifts. In the interest of saving lives and reducing suffering, medical technology serves the most basic of desires: that of self-preservation. Yet as philosopher Hadley Arkes has noted, science since Bacon's time has carried with it a deadly dynamic. In the context of a modern social matrix, "the interest in self-preservation would be detached from a concern for the moral terms of principle on which our lives would be preserved."

> *Science and technology are good gifts of God to sinful people, who are capable of discovering ways to misuse even the best gifts.*

The good life never can be defined only in terms of the longer life, or the easier life. What does it profit a man if he eliminates pain and extends life expectancy if the price of these benefits includes an evil surcharge?

Several years ago, in a report on the use of fetal tissue to cure Parkinson's disease, ABC Television science correspondent George Strait acknowledged that ethical issues surrounded the acquisition and use of the tissue. But, he reassured the audience, the practical benefits of these procedures surely outweighed any ethical questions that might be troubling people. This is the pragmatic logic technology has encouraged.

Philosopher-historian Eric Voegelin described modern culture as being gnostic. You remember Gnosticism taught that knowledge rather than faith was the means of salvation. Some Gnostics championed the pursuit of esoteric, occultic knowledge to escape the corruption of fleshly existence. But other Gnostics (whose descendants are among us) sought in knowledge the transformation of the world. This strain, revived in the early Renaissance, produced a fascination with disciplines such as

*Conservative Christians often betray their commitment to truth by their uncritical faith in technique.*

astrology (knowledge of the stars), alchemy (knowledge of the elements), and numerology (knowledge of the secret relationship between numeric attributes). As the mechanisms of the universe were mastered, man could overcome evil by eliminating limitations.

This Gnosticism infected modern science from the beginning. Christian ideas about a reasonable God and a reasonable creation offered a foundation for the rise of science. But the perennial quest for human autonomy, the knowledge to be like God, did not suddenly cease when the apple fell on Newton's noggin. The effects of an older fruit and an earlier fall wormed their way into the heart of science.

Perhaps because of a fear of appearing antimodern, American Christians have difficulty in acknowledging the temptations that accompany science. It is important to be grateful for the benefits of science and technology. But why is it that, with the exception of the work of Darwin and Freud, many evangelicals treat science and technology as unmixed blessings?

Perhaps the reason is tied in with ways in which evangelicalism is more influenced by our culture's assumptions than is often acknowledged. There is a deep vein of pragmatism in the ground on which institutions are built. If theologically dubious evangelistic techniques seem to work in increasing the number of "conversions," the practical benefits of these approaches surely outweigh any theological questions that might be troubling the more scrupulous among us.

Loving our neighbors obligates us to discover truly better things for truly better living. Science and technology can help us in that pursuit. But loving God requires that we think beyond the merely practical to see clearly the principles that should govern us in making those discoveries.

# The Eternal Weight of Glory

*Mike Malone*

Every time I find myself in the express line at the grocery store, I observe two things: One, the "express" line isn't what it claims to be, and two, there is a picture of Joan Rivers on the cover of at least one of the national tabloids. I am amazed that someone her age can look so youthful.

Joan Rivers isn't the only one laboring to beat the odds through an interminable sequence of face-lifts, tummy tucks, and mud masks. Channel surfers, I am told, find a plethora of exercise programs, talk shows, specials, and lengthy advertisements given to defending the body against the inevitable.

Death is an anomaly. It is not human; it is inhuman. As beings made in the image of God, designed to know and enjoy him forever, one of our central drives is to resist death, even as it makes its incremental and inexorable advance. It isn't what we were made for, and its intrusion is unnatural.

Because death is offensive to us, we seek to avoid it. That avoidance shows up in our language. People don't die, they pass away or go on to a better place. The finality of death is a vagary which we are ill-equipped to face.

Our culture responds by dodging this finality rather than facing it. We do all we can to keep the inevitable at arm's length. Those of us with resources enough invest in club memberships and medicinal responses of one kind or another.

While we naturally avoid death, we do so unwisely. Our world and our lives are poor and paltry. The fall has ravaged us. Because the beauty of the creation remains, and because we have this insatiable appetite for life, the brokenness of everything around us is difficult to embrace. But brokenness is what characterizes this life.

Against this backdrop the Bible offers wisdom which we desperately need: "Therefore we do not lose heart. Though outwardly we are wasting away, yet inwardly we are being renewed day by day. For our light and momentary troubles are achieving for us an eternal glory that far outweighs them all. So we fix our eyes not on what is seen, but on what is unseen. For what is seen is temporary, but what is unseen is eternal"(2 Cor. 4:16–18). The Bible gives a priority to the inner person, the soul, and our first concern should be the development of the soul.

> *The Bible gives a priority to the inner person, the soul, and our first concern should be the development of the soul.*

To say that the Bible places a priority on the soul is not to suggest that there is a denial of the goodness of the created order, the body, or the things related to both. The Bible teaches the goodness of all that God has made (Gen. 1:31). Furthermore, the so-called cultural mandate (Gen. 1:28) underlies the affirmation that all labor under God is godly labor. Hence, human sexuality, the gifts of food, drink, friendship, and the body, the efforts of the artist, the plumber, the doctor, or the gardener, are to be recognized as good gifts of God.

Also, to acknowledge that the outer man is wasting away does not open the door to self-determination. Dr. Jack Kevorkian is not God, and to arrogate to himself God's sole prerogative is the height not of compassion but of arrogance. God is the lord of life and death. He alone sets the limits of each. While terminal illness raises hard questions, whether to terminate life aggressively and premeditatedly is not one of them.

Our culture has things out of order. The preoccupation with the material world, specifically the body and its preservation, or the malicious destruction of the body when it no longer serves our purposes, will lead to the atrophy and death of the inner world of the soul. It is an idolatry, and idols always break the hearts of their worshipers.

We have not heeded our souls. As a result, life grows increasingly nasty, brutish, and boring. Attention to this established order of things will change life for us. We Christians should be preoccupied with our souls. In this preoccupation with the inner world, the world of the soul, the work of God will renew and transform us, and we will find life in the outer world to be more manageable and even lovely. Remember the opening words of Augustine's autobiography: "You have made us for Yourself, O God, and our hearts are restless until they rest in Thee." As the soul rests in God, life is found.

# For Reflection and Discussion

## Chapter 1: *Healing, Suffering, and the New Medicine*

1. Given the vast medical resources and advances of our time, what accounts for the transition in medicine from healing and the treatment of symptoms to killing and the relief of suffering?

2. Do you agree with Nigel Cameron's implication that the writing and use of "living wills" reflects this transition in medicine? However the question is answered, what might be a Christian perspective on living wills?

3. In what ways might doctors and pastors team to protect the interests of patients and parishioners who often are overshadowed by family members, insurance companies, and medical "experts"?

4. What contributed to the breakup of what Cameron calls "Christian Hippocratism" that mediated medical practice in the past?

5. Cameron calls for a renewal of the Christian Hippocratic vision. How could that grand heritage be rekindled within the

context of the modern health-care system? How, with an appeal to common grace, might Christian physicians work with unbelieving physicians who would share the same goal?

## Chapter 2: *Of Doctors and Other Priests*

1. Do you agree with Michael Beates's claim that we have lost the moral ability to accept death as our forefathers did? If so, how does that lost moral ability express itself, practically speaking, in modern life?

2. Beates encourages deliberation on life-and-death issues before families face a health crisis. In what ways can a family responsibly consider those issues before the circumstances are forced upon it?

3. What "benefits" of current medical practice, other than the harvesting of organs of aborted children, ought the Christian refuse when pressed to make a quick life-and-death decision?

4. What principles, other than preserving life as long as possible, stem from the biblical teaching that the believer's body is the temple of the Holy Spirit?

5. Scripture is filled with examples of how God transforms "deformities," "disabilities," and "handicaps" into assets, blessings, and wonders of grace. What does this pattern say about our current desire for perfection in people, our children, and ourselves?

## Chapter 3: *Death with Dignity: The "Right" to Die*

1. Harold Brown relates the "euthanasia wave" to the "abortion wave" that rolled twenty years before. What other "waves" have followed in the wake of abortion on demand?

2. In spite of the popularity of what Brown terms the euphemisms of "death with dignity" and "mercy killing," why do people avoid using the term *killing?*

3. How should the belief that human life is a prelude to an afterlife affect the way we view death? Specifically, why is mercy killing wrong if it provides an express route to the other side of eternity?

4. How is the practice of relieving or ending physical suffering through killing an expression of the current cultural enthronement of personal peace and affluence?

5. While generally not supportive of euthanasia or abortion, how do modern Christians worship at the altar of personal peace and affluence?

## Chapter 4: *The Right Questions*

1. Ken Myers suggests Christians often seek answers to the wrong questions. In addition to the examples he cites, what other right questions need to be raised in medical ethics?

2. How does one develop the intuition and ability, as Myers has done, to identify a wrong question and raise the right questions?

3. How do the structures of modern life reinforce the understanding of personhood as being an individual with rights rather than a member of society connected to a fabric of duties and responsibilities?

4. Do you agree with Myers that the Christian before God is better defined in terms of kinship than in abstract, ontological categories? If so, how does this relational definition affect biomedical ethics?

5. Myers contends "prudence" has been a neglected player in ethical questions. How does the neglect of "the best thing

to do" reap tragic consequences in life, and especially in medical ethics?

## Chapter 5: *Just Do Right*

1. Do you agree that life-and-death decisions are "agonizingly complex" and require more than "unswerving dogma"? Is more than what George Grant terms "unswerving valor" needed, and if so, what?

2. Why do people prefer the easy answers more than the right ones? What ultimately contributes to making life complex, whether in Paul's day or ours?

3. How can Christians resist the prevailing wisdom of the world?

4. Grant claims that Christians need to do more than advance a merely propositional message; they need the courage that wants to do right and knows how to do right. How then do we go about instilling that courage and ability?

## Chapter 6: *But Lord, My Lawyer Said It Would Be Okay*

1. Kenneth Connor argues that civil law, because it "follows rather than leads," is seldom an adequate guide to ethics. Is law ever an appropriate guide to ethics? When, for example, in recent United States history did changes in law lead to changes in behavior?

2. What accounts for the changes in the United States away from a law rooted in the transcendent values of Scripture?

3. Abraham Lincoln argued in reference to slavery that no one should have a legal right to do what is morally wrong. Does this mean that civil prohibitions need to cover every possible moral wrong? If not, what determines which moral wrongs

should be legally codified? How does Lincoln's initial desire to restrain the spread of slavery, rather than abolish it, fit into these considerations?

4. What drives today's current preoccupation with privacy and personal autonomy?

5. Connor refers to the numerous conflicts between current civil law and a "careful examination of Scripture on subjects relating to the sanctity of life, marriage, and the family." To what extent should Christians seek changes in civil codes to reflect more biblical standards?

## Chapter 7: *Utilitarianism and the Moral Life*

1. Do you agree with J. P. Moreland that utilitarianism is on the rise in our pragmatic culture, and if so, why? How would our society be different if utilitarianism were on the decline?

2. Moreland illustrates how utilitarianism can justify physician-assisted suicide and the abortion of unborn, deformed children. How does utilitarianism influence modern attitudes and practices concerning the whole issue of birth control?

3. Why do humans seem more concerned with the consequences of their actions than their inherent quality or character?

4. Are consequences of behavior ever a legitimate factor in ethics? Where do consequences fit into what Moreland terms virtue and deontological ethics?

5. To what extent do modern evangelicals reflect a utilitarian approach to the Christian life? How would evangelicals be different if they tempered that utilitarianism?

## Chapter 8: *An Unchanging Standard*

1. R. C. Sproul writes that modern technology has introduced ethical questions that historically have not been

addressed by Christians. Identify a few of those questions that relate, for example, to life-support systems and *in vitro* fertilization.

2. Sproul suggests "basic principles" are needed to address modern ethical concerns. What "clear and normative" principles does the author set forth as tools to help mediate medical ethics today? What other principles might be added to his list?

3. What is the relationship between law and ethics? Can civil law ever be framed to reflect ethical norms more than it does, and if so, how?

4. Why do men and women invoke "love" to justify behavior that often violates the expressed will of God?

5. How does the law of God reveal "what righteousness requires" in the complex ethical matters that Christians face today but were not contemplated by the writers of the Bible? What other subordinate sources of information and knowledge can legitimately inform the quest for discerning God's will?

## Chapter 9: *You Shall Not Be Gods*

1. A fine line separates the responsible, God-given exercise of dominion of the earth and man's reactive grasp for autonomy. Do you agree with R. C. Sproul's implication that sending a man to the moon crossed over that line, and if so, how?

2. How do we know when the application of technology represents the denial of God rather than an expression of proper stewardship?

3. What factors contributed to the nineteenth century being, in the words of Sproul, the second most peaceful century in history?

4. Do you agree that the Enlightenment is responsible for the horrors of the twentieth century? What other factors, if any, contributed to the tragedies of our time?

5. How can technology and science be harnessed for godly purposes?

## Chapter 10: *The Promise of Prozac and Silicone*

1. Why are Americans more concerned with physical health and outward appearance than spiritual health and inner character?

2. To what extent do the size, status, and dominance of the medical industry in the United States, when compared to the institutional church, reflect that inversion of values? In the mid-nineteenth century, why was the church more influential than today?

3. If Americans wake up from what Randy Crenshaw calls the "morning after" of American medicine to begin seeking after the promise of the Great Physician, how might that change our nation as well as our health?

4. In what practical ways can we develop and nurture our souls to build the inner strength, beauty, and character described in 1 Peter 3?

5. Crenshaw maintains that the six-year increase in life expectancy in our century is not remarkable. If life expectancy cannot be extended much further, does that mean its pursuit by doctors, researchers, and scientists is not a legitimate Christian endeavor? If not, how might a Christian professional redeem that field for Christ's kingdom?

## Chapter 11: *Prenatal Techniques*

1. Do you agree with the position of the Christian Medical and Dental Society on *in vitro* fertilization? What other conditions or prohibitions would you apply to the practice?

2. How does eugenics in general, and surrogate parenthood or *in vitro* fertilization with sperm or eggs from an unmarried

partner in particular, reflect and contribute to the weakening of marriage and family bonds? Even using sperm and eggs from husband and wife, does *in vitro* fertilization represent any threat to the marital bond?

3. Is bearing a child to provide an organ for a needy older sibling a questionable practice? Under what circumstances might you consider having a second child to save the life of your first?

4. Is the use of eugenics to influence the characteristics of one's progeny any different from the use of birth control to determine the quantity of one's progeny? To what extent does birth control reflect the same spirit that drives eugenics?

5. What does God's command in Genesis to "be fruitful and multiply" mean in the late twentieth century?

## Chapter 12: *The Human Body Shop*

1. What does the transition from appreciating the human body as a sacred creation to trading the human body as a secular commodity say about the church in Western society?

2. Is it too late to reverse the marketing and commercialization of the human body? If not, what opportunities exist to allow sanity and Christian values to shift gears away from this frightful and troubling trend?

3. How can the Christian community speak responsibly and convincingly against the trade of blood, organs, fetal life, reproductive systems, and genes?

4. What limitations have Christians placed upon themselves that hinder their ability to be taken seriously in the medical ethics debate? What could be done to lessen those limitations?

5. While the "Christian Right" has brought evangelicals into the political process, the deliberation of medical issues on the cutting edge is more often played out in the health professions,

academia, and the research community—arenas less influenced by direct action or public pressure. How should these institutional realities inform a Christian strategy of responding to what Andrew Kimbrell terms an ethical free fall?

## Chapter 13: *Can You Clone a Soul?*

1. Like they do with all good gifts, humans have a tendency to transform responsible care and use of the human body into worship. How does the Christian exercise proper stewardship of the body without falling into idolatry?

2. What is the relationship, if any, to the extension of life at all costs (a goal which may represent respect for life) to the harvesting of brain tissue from aborted babies (a means of extending life that devalues other human life)? What is responsible for these seemingly conflicting medical practices? Do the means undermine the goal?

3. While the extension of life often may require heroic efforts, at what point does the Christian allow providence to run its course and allow the body simply to die? Can extraordinary means to keep life in the body ever represent idolatry, and if so, when?

4. How could we emulate Puritan Richard Baxter today in the exercise and care of our souls?

## Chapter 14: *Technology and the New Gnosticism*

1. How do improved material surroundings delude us into thinking life is better? How can the Christian resist equating the good life with an easier or longer existence?

2. In what ways does modern science reflect what Ken Myers calls the "perennial quest for human autonomy, the knowledge to be like God"?

3. How can science be redeemed from the Gnosticism and quest for autonomy Myers claims has infected the discipline? What limits Christians in pioneering such an effort?

4. In addition to the reasons cited by Myers, why do evangelicals embrace science and technology as unmixed blessings?

5. To what extent is Myers correct in claiming "evangelicalism is more influenced by our culture's assumptions than is often acknowledged"? What prevents evangelicals from tempering their pragmatism with theological reflection?

## Chapter 15: *The Eternal Weight of Glory*

1. Why is death offensive to most people? Aside from terminology, how else is that offensiveness expressed in our culture?

2. How does the "central human drive to resist death" highlighted by Mike Malone relate to the "death with dignity" movement described by Harold Brown in chapter 3? Are the two contradictory or does some connection exist?

3. Malone says our culture prefers to dodge the finality of death rather than face it. If we faced death head-on, how would life be different? What does "facing it" mean?

4. Why is accepting the "brokenness" of life so hard for humans, including many Christians? What keeps us from coming to terms with this reality?

5. Malone claims if we shower our souls with the attention we shower on our bodies, "God will renew and transform us, and we will find life in the outer world to be more manageable and even lovely." What are the steps that could lead to the reversal of our priorities?